*"...to care for him who shall have borne the battle and for his widow, and his orphan..."*

*- Abraham Lincoln*

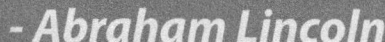

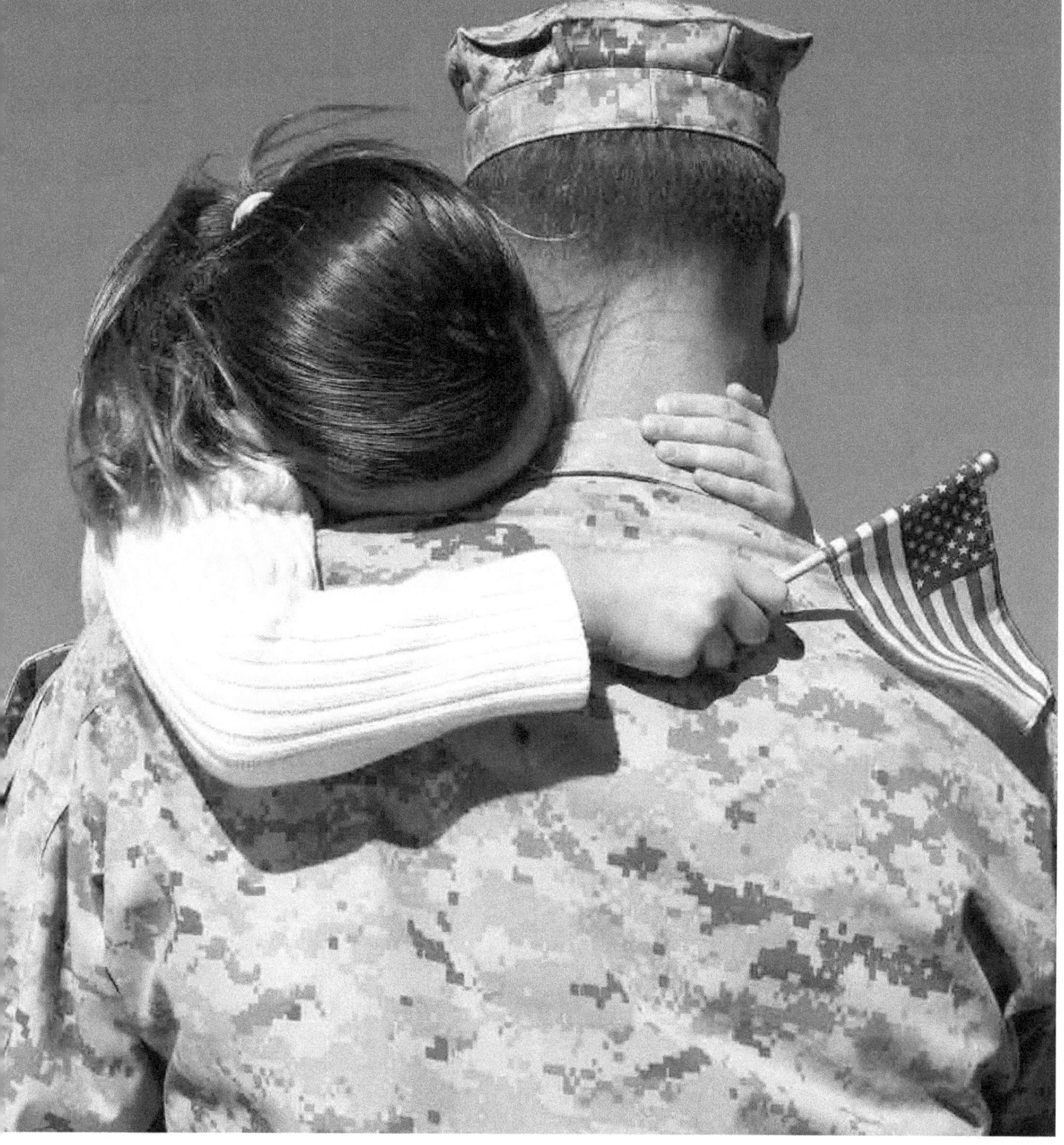

# Table of Contents

# Introduction

This guide is designed to provide Veterans and their families with the information they need to understand VA's health care system—eligibility requirements, the health benefits and services available to help Veterans and copays that certain Veterans may be charged.

Additionally, inside you will find helpful information about My HealtheVet, Creditable Coverage for Medicare Part D, Income Verification and medically related travel benefits.

This brochure is not intended to provide information on all of the health services offered by VA. If we have not addressed your specific questions, additional assistance is available at the following resources:

Your local VA health care facility's Enrollment Office
www.va.gov/healthbenefits
www.myhealth.va.gov
VA toll-free 1-877-222-VETS (8387) between the hours of 8:00 AM and 8:00 PM ET, Monday - Friday

> ## *VA enrollment also allows health care benefits to become completely portable throughout the entire VA system.*

## Overview

Today's Veterans have a comprehensive medical benefits package, which VA administers through an annual patient enrollment system. The enrollment system is based on priority groups to ensure health care benefits are readily available to all enrolled Veterans (see Enrollment Priority Groups on page 19).

Complementing the expansion of benefits and improved access is our ongoing commitment to providing the very best in quality service. Our goal is to ensure our patients receive the finest quality health care regardless of the treatment program, regardless of the location. In addition to our ongoing quality assurance activities, we've made it easier for Veterans to get the health care they need. New locations continue to be added to the VA health care system—bringing the total number of treatment sites to over 1,400 nationwide.

All Veterans—including those who have special eligibility—are encouraged to apply for enrollment. Enrollment helps us determine the number of potential Veterans who may seek VA health care services and is a very important part of our planning efforts.

Enrollment in the VA health care system provides Veterans with the assurance that comprehensive health care services will be available when and where they are needed during that enrollment period. In addition to the assurance that services will be available, enrolled Veterans welcome not having to repeat the application process—regardless of where they seek their care or how often.

## Veterans Choose the VA Facility

As part of the enrollment process, Veterans will be given the opportunity to select the VA health care facility or Community Based Outpatient Clinic (CBOC) to serve as his/her preferred facility.

# Benefits on the Go

VA enrollment also allows health care benefits to become completely portable throughout the entire VA health care system. Enrolled Veterans who are traveling or who spend time away from their preferred facility may obtain care at any VA health care facility across the country without the worry of having to reapply. Once you are enrolled, you will always be enrolled, however, you may be asked to update/verify your demographic and/or financial information when seeking care at a new VA facility. Veterans with a service-connected condition may receive treatment for that condition even in a foreign country (see Foreign Medical Program on page 26).

# Notice of Privacy Practices

Veterans who are enrolled for VA health care benefits have various privacy rights under federal law and regulations, including the right to a Notice of Privacy Practices. The VA Notice of Privacy Practices provides enrolled Veterans with information regarding how VHA may use and disclose personal health information, of their rights to know when and to whom their health information may have been disclosed, how to request access to or receive a copy of their health information on file with VHA, and how to request an amendment to correct inaccurate information on file and file a privacy complaint. The VA Notice of Privacy Practices may be obtained through the Internet at **www.va.gov/vhapublications/viewpublication.asp?pub_id=1089** or through the mail by writing the VHA Privacy Office (19F2), 810 Vermont Avenue NW, Washington, DC 20420.

# Your Personal VA Health Information Online

VA offers Veterans, Servicemembers, their dependents and caregivers their own Personal Health Record through My HealtheVet, found at **www.myhealth.va.gov**.

My HealtheVet's free, online Personal Health Record is available 24/7, wherever there is Internet access. If you are a VA patient and have an upgraded account (obtained by completing the one-time In-Person Authentication* process), you can:

- Participate in Secure Messaging with your participating VA health care team members
- View key portions of your DoD Military Service Information
- Get your VA Wellness Reminders
- View your VA Appointments
- View your VA Lab Results
- View your VA Allergies and Adverse Reactions
  - o PLUS, participate in future features as they become available

With My HealtheVet, you can access trusted health information to better manage your health care and learn about other VA benefits and services.

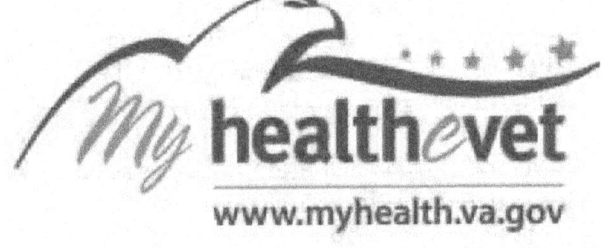

My Health, My Care: 24/7 Online Access to VA

My HealtheVet helps Veterans partner with your VA health care teams by providing tools to make shared, informed decisions. Simply follow the directions on the website to register. If you are a VA patient registered on My HealtheVet, you can begin to refill your VA medications online. You can also use the VA Blue Button to view, print, or download the health data currently in your My HealtheVet account. You can share this information with your family, caregivers or others such as your non-VA health care providers. It puts you in control of your information stored in My HealtheVet.

Accessible through My Health*e*Vet VA Blue Button also provides Veterans who were discharged from military service after 1979 access to your DoD Military Service Information.  This information may include Military Occupational Specialty (MOS) codes, pay details, service dates, deployment, and retirement periods.

*To access the advanced My Health*e*Vet features, Veterans will need to get an upgraded account by completing a one-time process at their VA facility called In-Person Authentication . Visit My Health*e*Vet at **www.myhealth.va.gov**, register and learn more about In-Person Authentication PLUS the many features and tools available to you 24/7 anywhere you have Internet access.

If you have any questions about My Health*e*Vet, contact the My Health*e*Vet Coordinator at your local VA facility.

## Frequently Asked Questions

### *Were there changes to allow more high income Veterans to enroll for VA health care?*

Yes.  On June 15, 2009, VA amended its regulations to expand enrollment of certain Veterans with higher income. Under this provision, VA is enrolling Priority Group 8 Veterans whose income does not exceed the new VA National Income Thresholds by more than 10%.  While this provision does not remove consideration of income, it does increase income thresholds.

### *Where can I find the new income thresholds?*

Because of the changes to the income thresholds each year, they are not published in this brochure.  However, the income threshold tables can be viewed on-line at
**http://www.va.gov/healthbenefits/cost/income_thresholds.asp**

### *How can I verify my enrollment?*

Once you enroll, you will receive either a letter or a newly introduced Veterans Health Benefits Handbook from us notifying you of the status of your enrollment.  You may also call us to verify your enrollment at 1-877-222-VETS (8387) between the hours of 8:00 AM and 8:00 PM ET, Monday - Friday.

**www.va.gov/healthbenefits/**

# Eligibility and Medical Program Benefits

## Basic Eligibility

If you served in the active military, naval or air service and are separated under any condition other than dishonorable, you may qualify for VA health care benefits. Current and former members of the Reserves or National Guard who were called to active duty (other than for training only) by a federal order and completed the full period for which they were called or ordered to active duty may be eligible for VA health care as well.

## Minimum Duty Requirements

Most Veterans who enlisted after September 7, 1980, or entered active duty after October 16, 1981, must have served 24 continuous months or the full period for which they were called to active duty in order to be eligible. This minimum duty requirement may not apply to Veterans who were discharged for a disability incurred or aggravated in the line of duty, discharged for a hardship, or received an "early out." Since there are a number of other exceptions to the minimum duty requirements, VA encourages all Veterans to apply in order to determine their enrollment eligibility.

## Women Veterans Eligibility

Current estimates of the projected growth of women Veterans predict there will be 1.9 million by 2020, up from 1.1 million in 1980. Thus, women will continue to make up a larger share of the Veteran population, add to its diversity, and require Veteran services geared to their specific needs.

VA is committed to meeting women Veterans' unique needs by delivering the highest quality health care in a setting that ensures privacy, dignity, and sensitivity. Your local VA facility offers a variety of services, including:

- Women's gender-specific health care (menopause evaluation and symptom management, osteoporosis, incontinence, birth control, breast and gynecological care, maternity and limited infertility services).

- Screening and disease prevention programs (for example, mammograms, bone density screening, and cervical cancer screening).

- Childbirth services to the newborn child of a woman Veteran

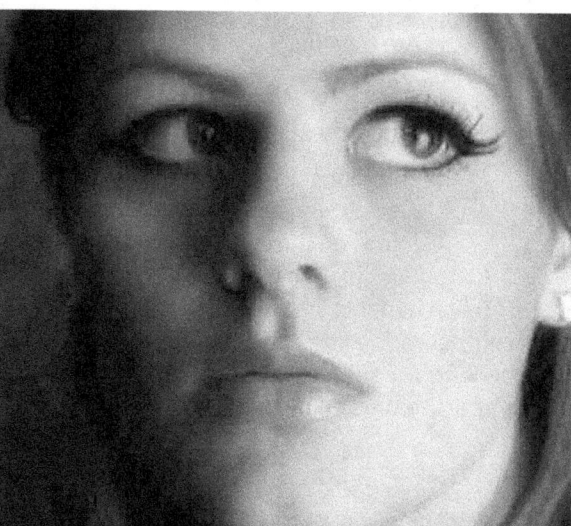

*Current estimates of the projected growth of women Veterans predict there will be 1.9 million by 2020, up from 1.1 million in 1980.*

Routine gynecologic services available through your local VA facility include:

- Human Papilloma Virus (HPV) vaccinations
- Pelvic exams, ultrasounds
- Birth control counseling and management (medical and surgical)
- Pre-pregnancy care
- Treatment and prevention of sexually transmitted infections

Your provider can assist with routine exams, diagnosis, and management of:

- Pelvic/abdominal pain
- Abnormal vaginal bleeding
- Vaginal symptoms (dryness/infections)
- Breast and other women's cancers
- Abnormal cervical screening results
- Infertility evaluation, including intrauterine insemination (IUI).  VA is not authorized to provide or cover the cost of in vitro fertilization (IVF).
- Sexual dysfunction

Female Veterans are potentially eligible for Fee Basis care.  However, the decision to utilize such care is left to the facility providing your care.  By law, Fee Basis care can only be provided when your treating facility cannot provide you the care you require or because of geographical inaccessibility

Contact your local Women Veterans Program Manager for more information on available services.

# Medically Related Travel Benefits

Veterans may qualify for mileage reimbursement if they fall into one of the following categories:

- Have a service-connected disability rating of 30 percent or more
- Are traveling for treatment of a service-connected condition
- Receive a VA pension
- Are traveling for a scheduled compensation or pension examination
- Does not have income that exceeds the maximum annual VA pension rate
- Veterans meeting the above conditions may also be provided special mode travel (e.g., wheelchair van, ambulance) based on a clinical determination of need (authorization is not required for emergencies if a delay would endanger their life or health).  More information on mileage rates and deductibles can be found on the internet at **www.va.gov/healthbenefits**

Travel benefits are subject to a deductible. Exceptions to the deductible requirement include: 1) travel for a compensation and pension examination; and 2) travel by an ambulance or a specially equipped van. Because travel benefits are subject to annual mileage rate and deductible changes, we publish a separate document detailing these amounts each year. You can obtain a copy at any VA health care facility.

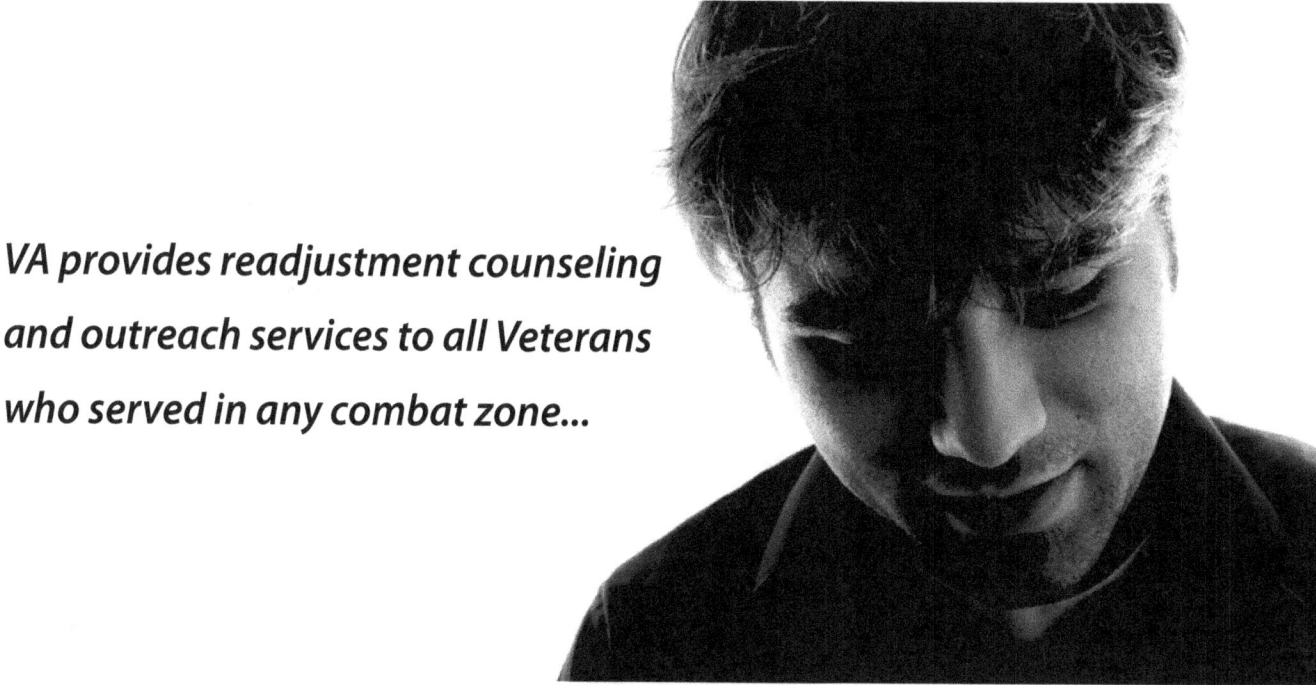

*VA provides readjustment counseling and outreach services to all Veterans who served in any combat zone...*

## Readjustment Counseling Services

VA provides readjustment counseling and outreach services to all Veterans who served in any combat zone, through community based counseling centers called Vet Centers. Services are also available for their family members for military related issues. Veterans have earned these benefits through their service and all are provided at no cost to the Veteran or family. The Vet Centers are staffed by small multidisciplinary teams of dedicated personnel, many of whom are combat Veterans themselves. Vet Center staffs are available toll-free during normal business hours at 1-800-905-4675 (Eastern) and 1-866-496-8838 (Pacific). For information online, visit **www.vetcenter.va.gov.**

## Veterans Crisis Line

The Veterans Crisis Line is a toll-free, confidential resource that connects Veterans in crisis and their families and friends with qualified, caring VA responders.

Veterans and their loved ones can call **1-800-273-8255** and **Press 1**, chat online at **www.VeteransCrisisLine.net** or send a text message to 838255 to receive free, confidential support 24 hours a day, 7 days a week, 365 days a year, even if they are not registered with VA or enrolled in VA health care.

The professionals at the Veterans Crisis Line are specially trained and experienced in helping Veterans of all ages and circumstances—from Veterans coping with mental health issues that were never addressed to recent Veterans struggling with relationships or the transition back to civilian life.

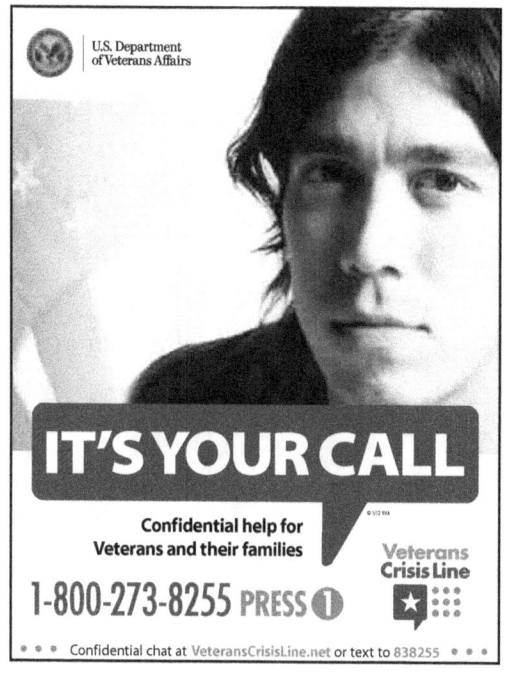

# National Call Center for Homeless Veterans

VA has founded a National Call Center for Homeless Veterans to ensure that homeless Veterans or Veterans at-risk for homelessness have free, 24/7 access to trained counselors. The hotline is intended to assist homeless Veterans and their families, VA Medical Facilities, federal, state and local partners, community agencies, service providers and others in the community. To be connected with a trained VA staff member call **1-877-4AID VET (877-424-3838)**.

- Call for yourself or someone else

- Free and confidential

- Trained VA counselors to assist

- Available 24 hours a day, 7 days a week

- We have information about VA homeless programs and mental health services in your area that can help you.

More information can be found at **www.va.gov/HOMELESS/NationalCallCenter.asp**.

# Family Caregivers Program

On May 5, 2010, Public Law 111-163, Caregivers and Veterans Omnibus Health Services Act of 2010 was signed into law. The purpose of the caregivers benefit program is to provide certain medical, travel, training, and financial benefits to caregivers of certain veterans and Servicemembers who were seriously injured during service on or after September 11, 2001. VA began accepting 10-10CG (Caregiver) applications on May 9, 2011. VA's Family Caregivers Program provides support and assistance to caregivers of post 9/11 Veterans and Service Members being medically discharged. Eligible primary Family Caregivers can receive a stipend, training, mental health services, travel and lodging reimbursement, and access to health insurance if they are not already under a health care plan. For more information, contact your local VA medical facility and speak with a Caregiver Support Coordinator, visit **www.caregiver.va.gov** or dial toll-free 1-855-260-3274.

# VA Health Care Enrollment

## Applying for Enrollment is Now Easier and Faster than ever...

No more signing the application or mailing it in...applying is now easier and faster than ever! We've even shortened the form to make it easier to apply. When applying online at **https://www.1010ez.med.va.gov/sec/vha/1010ez/**, Veterans simply fill out the application online and electronically submit it to VA for processing. No need for additional documents to verify military service - if the Veteran was recently discharged, we will get that information. Applying online significantly reduces the processing time for enrollment for Veterans to be able to access their medical benefits. Apply online now at **https://www.1010ez.med.va.gov/sec/vha/1010ez**. If you need help filling out the form while online, call 1-877-222-VETS (8387) between the hours of 8:00 AM and 8:00 PM ET, Monday - Friday, or click on the "chat online with representative" button located on the website and a representative will assist you.

The application form can be downloaded from the website above, or if you prefer, to complete the application over the phone, or have a paper copy mailed to you, you may do so by calling 1-877-222-VETS (8387) between the hours of 8:00 AM and 8:00 PM ET, Monday - Friday. You may also apply in person at any VA Healthcare Facility. Once you have submitted your application, you will be notified via letter of the status of your enrollment and priority group assignment.

Once you enroll in the VA health care system, you will receive either an enrollment letter or a Veterans Health Benefits Handbook. Each customized handbook includes VA health care benefit information, based on the Veteran's specific eligibility factors, in an organized, easy-to-read format. The handbook provides a current description of VA health care benefits available to each enrolled Veteran. It also includes information on the Veteran's preferred facility, copay responsibilities, how to schedule appointments, ways to communicate treatment needs, patient rights, how to obtain copies of medical records and more. For more information, visit **www.va.gov/healthbenefits/vhbh**.

*Regulations have enabled VA to relax income restrictions on enrollment for health benefits.*

## Priority Group 8 Enrollment Relaxation

Regulations went into effect on June 15, 2009 which enabled the Department of Veterans Affairs (VA) to relax income restrictions on enrollment for health benefits. While this provision does not remove consideration of income, it does increase income thresholds. You may be eligible for enrollment under this provision. The VA National Income Thresholds can be found online at **www.va.gov/healthbenefits/assets/documents/publications/AnnualThresholds.asp**.

Although the income relaxation regulation described above allows certain higher-income Veterans to be enrolled in the VA health care system, the previous Enrollment Restriction, effective January 17, 2003, by which VA suspended NEW enrollment of Veterans assigned to Priority Groups 8e and 8g is still in effect (VA's lowest priority group consisting of higher income Veterans). However, VA encourages Veterans in these priority groups to reapply for enrollment. They may now qualify if their current household income does not exceed the adjusted income thresholds under current regulations. The VA National Income Thresholds can be found on line at **www.va.gov/healthbenefits/assets/documents/publications/AnnualThresholds.asp**.

New Veteran applicants are assigned to Priority Groups 8e and 8g based on the following:

- The Veteran does not have any special qualifying eligibility, such as a compensable service-connected disability

- The Veteran's household income exceeds the current year adjusted VA income threshold and the adjusted geographic income threshold for the Veteran's residence

- Veterans who decline to provide their financial information

Veterans enrolled in Priority Groups 8a and 8c on or before January 16, 2003, remain enrolled and continue to be eligible for the full-range of VA health care benefits

Changes in VA's available resources may affect the number of priority groups VA can enroll in a given year. If that occurs, VA will publicize the enrollment changes and notify affected enrollees.

**IMPORTANT:** Veterans who may otherwise be ineligible for enrollment based on income may still be eligible based on a VA Catastrophically Disabled determination or due to loss of income or other economic factor by applying for a Hardship determination.  For further information please contact VA at 1-877-222-VETS (8387) between the hours of 8:00 AM and 8:00 PM ET, Monday - Friday.

# Obtaining an Appointment

You may request a doctor's appointment at the time you apply in person, or by checking 'yes' to the question asking if you want an appointment on the application for enrollment.  An appointment will be made with a VA doctor or provider and you will be notified via mail of the appointment.   If you need health care before your scheduled appointment, you may contact the Enrollment Coordinator, your clinic contact, Urgent Care Clinic or the Emergency Room at your local VA medical facility.

# Updating Your Information Using the  Automated Health Benefits Renewal Form

Already enrolled and need to update your information?  Enrolled Veterans may now automatically submit updates to their address, phone number, health insurance and financial information using the automated online VA Form 1010EZR, Health Benefits Renewal Form available at **www.1010ez.med.va.gov/sec/vha/1010ez/Form/1010ezr. pdf.**  If you need help filling out the form while online, you may call 1-877-222-VETS (8387) between the hours of 8:00 AM and 8:00 PM ET, Monday - Friday, or click on the "chat online with representative" button located on the website and a representative will assist you.

Veterans may update their information at any time - whenever their financial or personal information changes, by completing VA Form 10-10EZR. Submitting the information online is the fastest way to update information and no signature is required.  Other ways to update information are by phone at 1-877-222-VETS (8387) between the hours of 8:00 AM and 8:00 PM ET, Monday - Friday, by mail or in person.  If mailing the form, be sure to sign and date the form.

*Every VA medical center has a team ready to welcome OEF/OIF/OND Servicemembers and to help coordinate their care.*

## Special Eligibility and Coordination of Care for Combat Veterans Serving in Combat Theater After 11/11/1998– Returning Servicemembers (OEF/OIF/OND)

VA is ready to provide health care and other medical services to our nation's returning OEF/OIF/OND Servicemembers. Every VA medical center has a team ready to welcome OEF/OIF/OND Servicemembers and to help coordinate their care. For more information about the various programs available for recent returning service members, log on to the Returning Servicemembers web site at **http://www.oefoif.va.gov/VA_Help.asp**.

Veterans who served in a theater of combat operations also have special eligibility for VA health care. Under the "Combat Veteran" authority VA provides cost-free health care services and nursing home care for conditions possibly related to military service and enrollment in Priority Group 6 or higher for 5 years from the date of discharge or release from active duty, unless eligible for enrollment in a higher priority group to:

Combat Veterans who enroll with VA under this enhanced Combat Veteran authority will continue to be enrolled even after their enhanced eligibility period ends, although they may be shifted to Priority Group 7 or 8, depending on their income level, and required to make applicable copays. Additionally, for care not related to combat service, copays may be required depending on their financial assessment and other special eligibility factors.

**NOTE: The 5-year enrollment period applicable to these Veterans begins on the discharge or separation date** of the service member from active duty military service, or in the case of multiple call-ups, the most recent discharge date.

## Financial Assessment (Means Testing) and Income Thresholds

While many Veterans qualify for enrollment and cost-free health care services based on a compensable service-connected condition or other qualifying factors, certain Veterans will be asked to complete a financial assessment, or means test as part of their initial enrollment application process to determine their eligibility for cost-free medications and travel benefits. Otherwise known as the Means Test, this financial information may be used to determine the applicant's enrollment priority group (see Enrollment Priority Groups section on page 19) and whether he/she is eligible for cost-free VA health care. Higher-income Veterans may be required to share in the expense of their care by paying copays (Refer to the Copay section of this booklet on page 21).

Veterans who are already enrolled may submit their subsequent annual means test or at anytime their income or demographic information changes using the automated Online 10-10EZR, Health Benefits Renewal Form, (see information on page 10).

Income threshold information can be found online at: **http://www.va.gov/healthbenefits/cost/income_ thresholds.asp** or you may contact the Enrollment Coordinator at your local medical facility.

Due to VA's restricting enrollment of Priority Groups 8e and 8g, Veterans applying for enrollment who do not have any other special eligibility qualifying factors and decline to provide financial information, may not be accepted for enrollment.

## Geographically-Based Copays

Recognizing the cost of living can vary significantly from one geographic area to another, Congress added income thresholds based on geographic locations to the existing VA national income thresholds (**www.va.gov/healthbenefits/cost/income_thresholds.asp**) for financial assessment purposes. This assists lower-income Veterans who live in high-cost areas by providing an enhanced enrollment priority and reducing the amount of their required inpatient copay.

Geographically-based copay reductions apply ONLY to INPATIENT SERVICES. Outpatient services, long-term care, as well as medication copays are NOT affected by this provision.

*Congress added income thresholds based on geographic locations to the existing VA national income thresholds for financial assessment purposes.*

## Catastrophically Disabled

To be considered catastrophically disabled, Veterans must have a severely disabling injury, disorder or disease that permanently compromises their ability to carry out the activities of daily living. The disability must be of such a degree that Veterans require personal or mechanical assistance to leave home or bed, or require constant supervision to avoid physical harm to themselves or others. Veterans may request a catastrophic disability evaluation by contacting the Enrollment Coordinator at their local VA health care facility. VA will make every effort to schedule an evaluation within 30 days of the request and there is no charge for the Catastrophic Disability evaluation. Veterans determined by a VA provider to be catastrophically disabled will be upgraded to Priority Group 4 if not otherwise eligible for a higher priority group. In addition, Veterans who are determined by VA to be Catastrophically Disabled receive cost-free care for their outpatient/inpatient treatment and for their medications. However, Veterans in this category may be subject to copays for extended care (long-term care).

NOTE: A Veteran who may not be eligible for enrollment due to VA's current enrollment restriction will be enrolled in Priority Group 4 if found to be Catastrophically Disabled.

## Income Verification

Veterans Health Administration's Income Verification (IV) program verifies earned and unearned total gross household income (spouse and dependents, if any) provided by non service-connected Veterans and Veterans rated non-compensable 0% service-connected.

The financial assessment is based on the Veteran's previous year gross household income (spouse and dependents, if any) and is used to determine their eligibility for VA health care benefits and in many cases, their priority group assignment. Income information provided by the Veteran is verified by matching records from the Internal Revenue Service and the Social Security Administration.

If the IV process confirms the Veteran's household income exceeds the established VA national income (means test) thresholds, the Veteran may be determined responsible for copays for health care provided since the date of completion of the initial financial assessment. In addition, if the Veteran enrolled on or after January 17, 2003, the Veteran's enrollment could become denied. As a result, the Veteran would no longer be eligible for VA health care for treatment of their non service-connected conditions. (For more information, refer to the Enrollment Restriction section on page 9 of this booklet or log on to **www.va.gov/healthbenefits/cost/financial_assessment.asp**).

# Financial Hardships

If you are a Veteran who is suffering from financial distress, struggling to pay your VA copays, lost your job or currently face a significant decrease in your household income, VA has programs that can assist you. Additionally, VA's Medical Care Hardship program could help Veterans qualify for VA enrollment for health care services if they had a recent change in their income, even if they were previously denied enrollment based on their household income. Veterans who have not applied for VA enrollment because they thought their income was too high may want to reconsider applying if their projected current year's income is lower. Hardship determinations may be approved if the Veteran's current year income is substantially reduced from the prior year. Personal circumstances, such as loss of employment, sudden decrease in income or increases in out-of-pocket Veteran or family health care expenses, factor into VA's hardship determination.

If you are a Veteran and unable to pay your copay charges, you should discuss the matter with the Revenue Office at the VA health care facility where you received your care.

**You must contact the facility where you received the care to request one of these options or call VA at 1-877-222-VETS (8387) between the hours of 8:00 AM and 8:00 PM ET, Monday - Friday.**

| Four possible options for Veterans unable to pay assessed copay charges | |
|---|---|
| **Hardship Determination** | If a Veteran's current year income is substantially reduced from the prior year, the Veteran may be eligible for exemption from medical and hospital care copays for a determined period of time (See your local Enrollment Coordinator for Hardship consideration). |
| **Waiver** | If there has been a significant change in income or significant expenses for medical care for Veteran or other family members, funeral arrangements or Veteran educational expenses. Waiver is for past debts only. See your local Revenue staff for additional information |
| **Offer in Compromise** | Offer for past debts only and acceptance of a partial payment in settlement and full satisfaction of debt. See your local Revenue staff for additional information |
| **Repayment Plans** | Payment of past debt over a period of 36 months. See your local Revenue staff for additional information |

# Veterans Identification Card

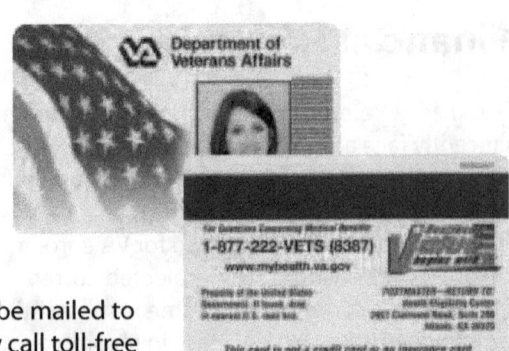

VA provides eligible Veterans a Veterans Identification Card (VIC) for use at VA health care facilities. This card provides quick access to VA health benefits. VA recommends all enrolled Veterans obtain a card.

Veterans may have their photo taken at their local VA health care facility. Once the Veteran's enrollment has been verified, the card will be mailed to the Veteran's mailing address, usually within 5 to 7 days. Veterans may call toll-free 1-877-222-VETS (8387) to check on the status of their card. In the event the card is lost or destroyed, a replacement card may be requested by contacting the VA where the picture was taken.

**NOTE:** VICs cannot be used as a credit or an insurance card and it does not authorize or pay for care at non-VA facilities.

The VIC does not contain any sensitive, identifying information such as the Veteran's Social Security number or date of birth on the face of the card. However, that information is coded into the magnetic stripe and barcode. For that reason, VA recommends that Veterans safeguard their VIC as they would a credit card.

# Private Health Insurance

Since many Veterans are medically co-managed by both VA and their local provider, VA encourages Veterans to retain any health care coverage they may already have—especially those in the lower enrollment priority groups described on pages 19 and 20, Enrollment Priority Groups. Veterans with private health insurance may choose to use these sources of coverage as a supplement to their VA benefits. It is important to note that VA health care is NOT considered a health insurance plan.

By law, VA is obligated to bill health insurance carriers for services provided to treat a Veteran's nonservice-connected conditions. Veterans are asked to cooperate by disclosing all relevant health insurance information. Eligible Veterans are not responsible for payment of VA medical services billed to their health insurance company that are not paid by their insurance carrier.

To ensure current insurance information is on file—including coverage through the Veteran's spouse—VA staff ensures that Veterans' health insurance information is updated during each visit. Identification of insurance information is essential to VA because collections received from insurance companies help supplement the funding available to provide services to Veterans. Veterans may now update any changes in their insurance by using the online Health Benefits Renewal (1010-EZR) form at **www.1010ez.med.va.gov/sec/vha/1010ez/Form/1010ezr.pdf**.

*...VA encourages Veterans to retain any health care coverage they may already have...*

| CAUTION! |
|---|
| Before cancelling health insurance coverage, enrolled Veterans should carefully consider the risks. |
| • There is no guarantee that in subsequent years Congress will appropriate sufficient funds for VA to provide care for all enrollment priority groups. |
| • Non-Veteran spouses and other family members generally do not qualify for VA health care. |
| • If participation in Medicare Part B is cancelled, it cannot be reinstated until January of the next year, and there may be a penalty for the reinstatement. |
| • Additional coverage for those Veterans that are medically co-managed by both VA and their local provider. |

## Insurance Collections

Since 1986, Veterans' health care services have been supplemented by funds collected from private health insurance companies. This supplement has allowed VA to provide services to numerous additional Veterans.

## Medicare Part D Prescription Drug Coverage/Creditable Coverage

If you are eligible for Medicare Part D prescription drug coverage, you need to know that enrollment in the VA health care system is considered **creditable coverage** for Medicare Part D purposes. This means that VA prescription drug coverage is at least as good as the Medicare Part D coverage. Since only Veterans may enroll in the VA health care system, dependents and family members do not receive credible coverage under the Veteran's enrollment.

However, there is one significant area in which VA health care is NOT creditable coverage: Medicare Part B (outpatient health care, including doctors' fees). Creditable coverage for Medicare Part B can only be provided through an **employer**. As a result, VA health care benefits to Veterans are not creditable coverage for the Part B program. So although a Veteran may avoid the late enrollment penalty for Medicare Part D by citing VA health care enrollment, that enrollment would not help the Veteran avoid the late enrollment penalty for Part B.

VA does not recommend Veterans cancel or decline coverage in Medicare (or other health care or insurance programs) solely because they are enrolled in VA health care. Unlike Medicare, which offers the same benefits for all enrollees, VA assigns enrollees to enrollment priority groups, based on a variety of eligibility factors, such as service-connection and income. There is no guarantee that in subsequent years Congress will appropriate sufficient medical care funds for VA to provide care for all enrollment priority groups. This could leave Veterans, especially those enrolled in one of the lower-priority groups, with no access to VA health care coverage. For this reason, having a secondary source of coverage may be in the Veteran's best interest.

In addition, a Veteran may want to consider the flexibility afforded by enrolling in both VA and Medicare. For example, Veterans enrolled in both programs would have access to non-VA physicians (under Medicare Part A or Part B) or may obtain prescription drugs not on the VA formulary if prescribed by non-VA physicians and filled at their local retail pharmacies (under Medicare Part D).

Additional information on Medicare Part D prescription drug coverage can be found online at the Health and Human Services Medicare website at **www.medicare.gov**.

*...a Veteran may want to consider the flexibility afforded by enrolling in both VA and Medicare.*

## Frequently Asked Questions

### *Must I reapply every year, and will I receive an enrollment confirmation?*

Depending on your priority group and the availability of funds for VA to provide health benefits to all enrollees, your enrollment will be automatically renewed without any action on your part. Veterans, based on their financial status, who are exempted from paying medical care copays or who are eligible for a reduced inpatient copay are required to update their financial information on an annual basis or when their income changes, using VA Form 10-10EZR. Should there be any change to your enrollment status, you will be notified in writing.

### *Can I request a Veterans Identification Card and/or an appointment before my enrollment is confirmed?*

Yes. If you are applying in person at any VA medical center, you can have your picture taken for the Veterans Identification Card and/or request an appointment for medical care at the same time you apply for enrollment. Additionally, you can indicate on the VA Form 10-10EZ if you desire an appointment and when your application is processed at the medical center, an appointment will be scheduled for you. You will be notified in writing of the appointment and your eligibility for medical care. Once your enrollment has been verified the identification card will be mailed to you, usually in 5-7 days after your enrollment has been verified. For Veterans 50% or more disabled from service-connected conditions and Veterans requesting care for a service-connected disability, those appointments have a higher priority (see Enrollment Priority Groups on pages 19 - 20) and will be scheduled within 30 days of the desired date. Veterans may be seen at VA facilities for emergency care while pending verification.

### *What if I cannot keep an appointment?*

VA asks that you help us provide timely service. If you cannot keep your appointment, please notify your facility as soon as possible so they can schedule another appointment for you, and use your cancelled appointment slot for another Veteran.

### *If enrolled, must I use VA as my exclusive health care provider?*

There is no requirement that VA become your exclusive provider of care. If you are a Veteran who is receiving care from both a VA provider and a private community provider, it is important for your health and safety that your care from both providers is coordinated, resulting in one treatment plan (co-managed care). Please be aware that our authority to pay for non-VA care is extremely limited (see pages 28 and 29). You may, however, elect to use your private health insurance benefits as a supplement for your VA health care benefits.

### *I am moving to another state. How do I transfer my care to a new VA health care facility?*

If you want to transfer your care from one VA health care facility to another, contact the Enrollment Office for assistance in transferring your records and establishing a new appointment.

### *How do I choose a preferred facility? How do I change my preferred facility?*

When you enroll, you will be asked to choose a preferred VA facility. This will be the VA facility where you will receive your primary care. You may select any VA facility that is convenient for you. If the facility you choose cannot provide the health care that you need, VA will make other arrangements for your care, based on administrative eligibility and medical necessity. If you do not choose a preferred facility, VA will choose the facility that is closest to your home.

You may change your preferred facility at any time. Simply discuss this with your primary care doctor. Your primary care doctor will coordinate your request with the Veterans Service Center at your local health care facility and make the change for you.

## What income is counted for the Financial Assessment (Means Test) & is family size considered?

VA considers your previous calendar year's gross household income and net worth. This includes the earned and unearned income and net worth of your spouse and dependent(s). Earned income is usually wages you receive from working. Unearned income can be interest earned, dividends received, money from retirement funds, Social Security payments, annuities or earnings from other assets. The number of persons in your family will be factored into the calculation to determine the applicable income threshold—both the VA national income threshold and the income threshold for your geographic region.

## What is a geographic income threshold?

By law, VA is required to identify Veterans who are required to defray the cost of medical care. Those Veterans whose income falls between the VA means test limits and the VA national geographic income threshold for the Veteran's locale will have their inpatient medical care copays reduced by 80%.

## For those Veterans who have more than one residence, which address is used for means testing under the geographically-based income thresholds?

The address used to determine your geographically-based income threshold is your permanent address and typically is the location where you declare residency for voting and tax purposes. To view geographic income thresholds, visit **http://www.va.gov/healthbenefits/cost/income_thresholds.asp.**

## How frequently are the VA national income thresholds updated?

VA national income thresholds, used for the Financial Assessment as well as for geographic adjustments for high cost-of-living areas, are updated annually. To view the current income thresholds, visit **http://www.va.gov/healthbenefits/cost/income_thresholds.asp.**

## Does Income Verification have access to my income tax return?

No, VA does not have access to your tax return. The Internal Revenue Service (IRS) and the Social Security Administration (SSA) share earned and unearned income data reported by employers and financial institutions.

## As a combat Veteran, will I be required to provide financial information and be billed?

No. Combat Veterans are not required to provide their financial information to determine their enrollment priority. However, they are encouraged to complete a financial assessment to determine if they may be exempt from copays for care or medications unrelated to their combat service or to establish beneficiary travel eligibility.

## If I decline to provide income and agree to make copays, will you still verify my income?

No, if you have agreed to make copays for care, you are not required to provide your income information, and we will not make any further attempts to verify your income for that year. However, Veterans who have no special eligibility and decline to provide income information are denied enrollment.

## What happens if at the end of the process my income is verified to be higher than the income thresholds?

Your copay status will be changed from copay exempt to copay required. VA facilities involved in your care will be notified of your change in status and to initiate billing for services provided during that income year. Your enrollment priority status may be changed if your financial status is adjusted by the income verification (IV) process. If your enrollment status is changed, you will be notified by mail.

## What if I receive a bill and cannot pay?

If you are unable to pay your bill, you should discuss the matter with the Revenue Office at the VA health care facility where you received your care.  There are four possible options that may be available to you

**Hardship Determination** – If a Veteran's current year income is substantially reduced from the prior year. Future exemption from medical and hospital care copays for a determined period of time.  (Must see Enrollment Coordinator for Hardship consideration.)

**Waiver** – If there has been a significant change in income or significant expenses for medical care for the Veteran or other family members, funeral arrangements or Veteran educational expenses.  Waiver is for past debts only. See your local revenue staff for additional information

**Offer in Compromise** – Offer for past debts only and acceptance of a partial payment in settlement and full satisfaction of debt.  See your local revenue staff for additional information

**Repayment Plans** – Payment of past debt generally over a period of 36 months.  See your local revenue staff for additional information

You must contact the facility at which you received the care to request one of these options

## What is a VA service-connected rating, and how do I establish one?

A service-connected rating is an official ruling by a Veterans Benefits Administration Regional Office that your illness or condition is directly related to your active military service. VA Regional Offices are also responsible for administering educational benefits, vocational rehabilitation and other benefit programs, including home loans. To obtain more information or to apply for any of these benefits, contact your nearest VA Regional Office at 1-800-827-1000 or visit us online at **www.va.gov**.

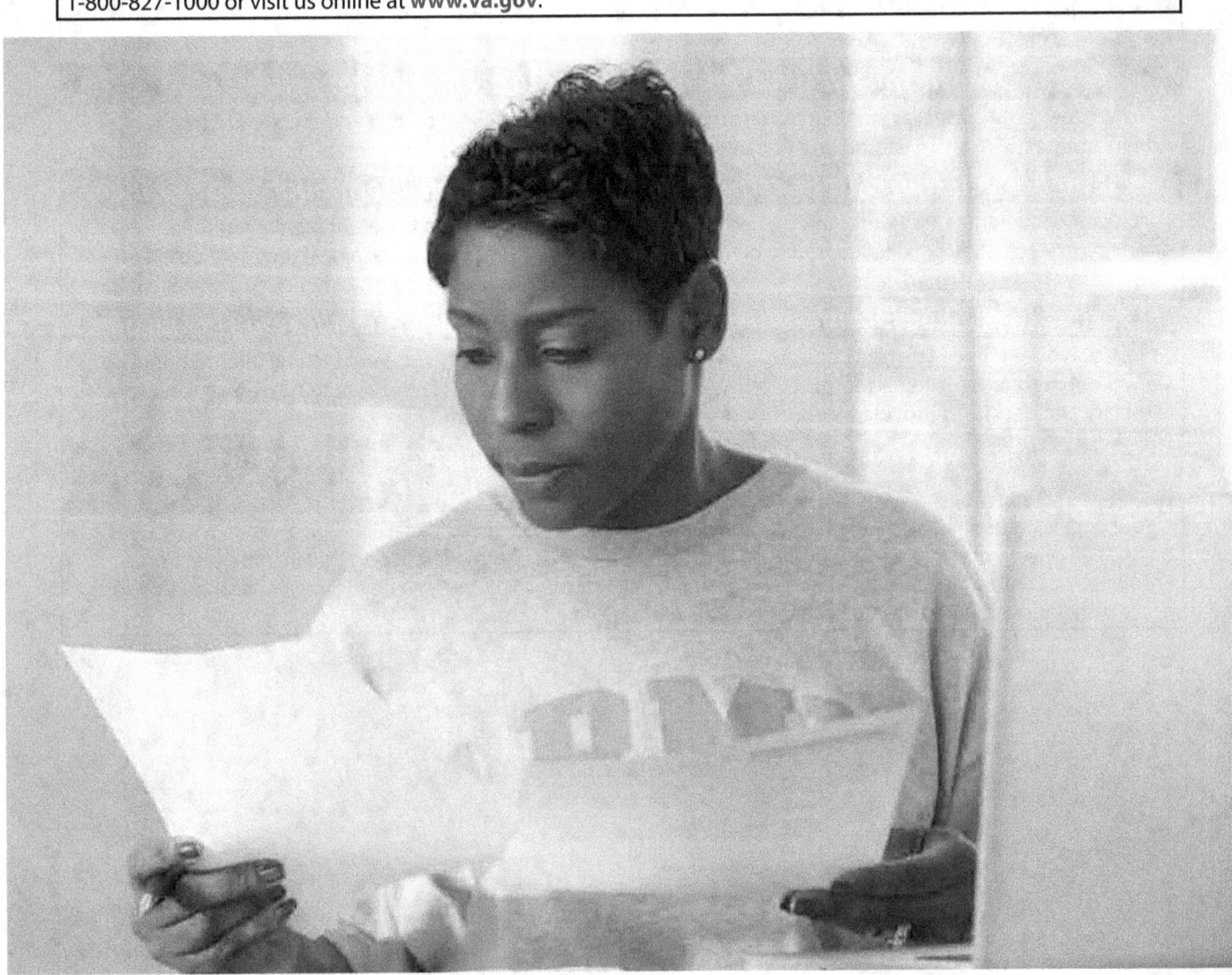

# VA Health Care Enrollment Priority Groups

Upon receipt of a completed application, the Veteran's eligibility will be verified. Based on his/her specific eligibility status, he/she will be assigned to one of the following priority groups. The priority groups range from 1 through 8 with Priority Group 1 being the highest priority and Priority Group 8 the lowest.

## Priority Group 1

| | |
|---|---|
| Veterans with service-connected disabilities 50% or more disabling | Veterans determined by VA to be unemployable due to VA service-connected conditions |

## Priority Group 2

| |
|---|
| Veterans with VA service-connected disabilities 30% or 40% disabling |

## Priority Group 3

| | |
|---|---|
| Veterans who are Former Prisoners of War (POWs) | Veterans awarded a Purple Heart medal |
| Veterans awarded the Medal of Honor (MOH) | Veterans whose discharge was for a disability that was incurred or aggravated in the line of duty |
| Veterans with VA service-connected disabilities 10% or 20% disabling | Veterans awarded special eligibility classification under Title 38, U.S.C., Section 1151, "benefits for individuals disabled by treatment or vocational rehabilitation" |

## Priority Group 4

| | |
|---|---|
| Veterans who are receiving aid and attendance or housebound benefits from VA | Veterans who have been determined by VA to be catastrophically disabled |

## Priority Group 5

| | |
|---|---|
| Non service-connected Veterans and noncompensable service-connected Veterans rated 0% disabled by VA with annual income and/or net worth below the VA national income threshold and geographically-adjusted income threshold for their resident location | Veterans receiving VA pension benefits |
| Veterans eligible for Medicaid programs | |

## Priority Group 6

| | |
|---|---|
| Veterans who served in the Republic of Vietnam between January 9, 1962 and May 7, 1975. | Veterans who served in the Southwest Asia theater of operations from August 2, 1990 through November 11, 1998. |

| Compensable 0% service-connected Veterans | Veterans exposed to ionizing radiation during atmospheric testing or during the occupation of Hiroshima and Nagasaki |
| --- | --- |
| Project 112/SHAD participants | |

| Veterans who served in a theater of combat operations after November 11, 1998, as follows: |
| --- |
| • Currently enrolled Veterans and new enrollees for five years post discharge |
| **Note:** After 5 years, Veterans will be assigned to the highest Priority Group they qualify for.. |

## Priority Group 7

Veterans with gross income above the VA national income threshold, and below the geographically-adjusted income threshold (GMT) for their resident location and who agree to pay copays

## Priority Group 8

Veterans with gross household income above the VA national income threshold and the geographically-adjusted income threshold for their residence location and who agree to pay copays

| **Veterans eligible for enrollment:** Noncompensable 0% service-connected and: | **Veterans eligible for enrollment:** Nonservice-connected and: |
| --- | --- |
| • Subpriority a: Enrolled as of January 16, 2003, and who have remained enrolled since that date and/or placed in this subpriority due to changed eligibility status<br>• Subpriority b: Enrolled on or after June 15, 2009 whose income exceeds the current VA National Income Thresholds or VA National Geographic Income Thresholds by 10% or less | • Subpriority c: Enrolled as of January 16, 2003, and who have remained enrolled since that date and/or placed in this subpriority due to changed eligibility status<br>• Subpriority d: Enrolled on or after June 15, 2009 whose income exceeds the current VA National Income Thresholds or VA National Geographic Income Thresholds by 10% or less |

| **Veterans not eligible for enrollment:** Veterans not meeting the criteria above: |
| --- |
| • Subpriority e: Noncompensable 0% service-connected<br>• Subpriority g: Nonservice-connected |

# Copays

While many Veterans qualify for cost-free health care services based on a compensable service-connected condition or other qualifying factors, most Veterans are asked to complete an annual financial assessment, to determine if they qualify for cost-free services. Veterans whose income exceeds the established income threshold as well as those who choose not to complete the financial assessment must agree to pay required copays to be eligible for VA health care services.

## Types of Copays

### Outpatient Copays* —
**based on the highest of two levels of service on any individual day.**

**Primary Care Services** – Services provided in a primary care setting to address overall patient care

**Specialty Care Services** – Services provided in Specialty Care area such as:

| | |
|---|---|
| Surgery | Radiology |
| Audiology | Optometry |
| Cardiology | |

and specialty tests such as:

| | |
|---|---|
| magnetic resonance imagery (MRI) | computerized axial tomography (CAT) scan |
| nuclear medicine studies (highest level of service) | |

*There is no copay requirement for preventive care services such as screenings or immunizations.*

### Medication Copays* —
**applicable to each prescription, including each 30-day supply or less of maintenance medications.**

*Includes an annual cap for enrollment priority groups 2 through 6.*

### Inpatient Copays —
**in addition to a standard copay charge for each 90 days of care within a 365 day period regardless of the level of service (such as intensive care, surgical care or general medical care); a per diem (daily) charge will be assessed for each day of hospitalization.**

# Long-Term Care Copays* —
## based on three levels of care (see Long-Term Care Benefits on page 31 for definitions).

| Community Living Centers (Nursing Home) Care/Inpatient Respite Care/Geriatric Evaluation | Adult Day Health Care/Outpatient Geriatric Evaluation/Outpatient Respite Care |
|---|---|
| Domiciliary Care | |

*Copays for Long-Term Care services start on the 22nd day of care during any 12-month period—there is no copay requirement for the first 21 days. Actual copay charges will vary from Veteran to Veteran depending on financial information submitted on VA Form 10-10EC.*

**NOTE:** There are no copays for hospice care provided in any setting.

## Outpatient Copays

**Primary Care Services** – services provided by a primary care clinician–$15

**Specialty Care Services** – In general, services delivered in a specialty outpatient clinic provided by highly-specialized, narrowly-focused health care professionals-services provided by a clinical specialist–Specialty Copay -$50

## Inpatient Copays

There are two inpatient copay rates – the full rate and the reduced rate. The reduced inpatient copay rate, which is 80% of the full inpatient rate, applies to Veterans meeting specific income requirements. Both the full inpatient copay rate and the reduced inpatient copay rate are computed over a 365 - day period. Because the Inpatient Copay rates change each year, they are published separately and can be found on line at **www.va.gov/healthbenefits/cost/copays.asp** or contact VA at 1-877-222-VETS (8387) between the hours of 8:00 AM and 8:00 PM ET, Monday - Friday for more information.

Recognizing that the cost of living can vary significantly from one geographic area to another, Veterans living in high cost areas may qualify for a reduced inpatient copay rate. Because the GMT copay rates change each year, they are published separately at **www.va.gov/healthbenefits/cost/copays.asp.**, or contact VA at 1-877-222-VETS (8387) for more information.

## Medication Copays

Currently, there is a $8 copay (subject to change) for each 30-day or less supply of medication provided on an outpatient basis for treatment of a non-service-connected condition for Veterans in Priority Group 2 through 6, with an annual copayment cap of $960, unless otherwise exempted. This copay is $9 for Veterans in Priority Group 7 or 8 with no annual copayment cap.

## Long Term Care Copays

Long term care copay are based on three levels of care

| | |
|---|---|
| | Up to $97 per day (Nursing Home, Respite, Geriatric Evaluation) |
| | $15 per day (Adult Day Health Care, Respite, Geriatric Evaluation) |
| | $5 per day |

## What is the copay for a 90-day supply of medication?

Even though a prescription may be written for 90 days, each 30-day or less supply is subject to that year's applicable medication copay rate. A 90-day supply would cost three times the applicable medication copay rate based on your Priority Group.

## Annual Changes to Copay Rates

Because the copay rates may change annually—including the annual cap on medication copays—they are published separately. Current year rates can be obtained at any VA health care facility or on the eligibility page on our Web site **http://www.va.gov/healthbenefits/assets/documents/publications/IB10-430.pdf.**

# Which Veterans Are Not Required to Make Copays?

**Many Veterans qualify for cost-free health care and/or medications based on:**

- Purple Heart recipient (may take copay test to determine medication copay status)

- Former Prisoner of War Status, or (both are cost-free)

- 50% or more Compensable VA service-connected disabilities, (0-40% service-connected may take co-pay test to determine medication copay status) or

- Veterans deemed catastrophically disabled by a VA provider

- Veterans with income below the income threshold

- Other qualifying factors, including treatment related to their military service experience.

**Some of the Services Exempt from Inpatient and Outpatient Copays**

- Special registry examinations offered by VA to evaluate possible health risks associated with military service

- Counseling and care for military sexual trauma

- Compensation and pension examinations are requested by the Veterans Benefits Administration (VBA). This is a physical exam to determine service-related illness or injuries for determination of a Veteran's entitlement to compensation and pension benefits.

- Care that is part of a VA-approved research project

- Care related to a VA-rated service-connected disability

- Readjustment counseling and related mental health services

- Care for cancer of head or neck caused by nose or throat radium treatments received while in the military

- Catastrophic Disability Exam

- Individual or Group Smoking Cessation or Weight Reduction services

- Publicly announced VA public health initiatives, for example, health fairs

- Care potentially related to combat service for Veterans that served in a theater of combat operations after November 11, 1998. This benefit is effective for 5 years after the date of Veteran's most recent discharge from active duty.

- Laboratory and electrocardiograms

- Hospice care

# Frequently Asked Questions

## *I am a recently discharged combat Veteran. Must I pay VA copays?*

If the services are provided for the treatment of a condition that may be potentially related to your military service in a theater of combat operations, you will not be charged any copays. Combat Veterans have an enhanced enrollment health benefit period of five years from their most recent discharge from active duty.

Veterans who qualify under this special eligibility are not subject to copays for conditions potentially related to their combat service. However, unless otherwise exempted, combat Veterans must either disclose their prior year gross household income OR decline to provide their financial information and agree to make applicable copays for care or services VA determines are clearly unrelated to their military service.

## *How many copay charges may be assessed during a single day?*

Veterans may be charged no more than one outpatient copay per day, regardless of the number of health care providers seen in a single day. The amount of the outpatient copay will be based on the highest level of service received that day. For example, if the Veteran has a specialty care visit and a primary care visit on the same day, the Veteran will be charged only for the specialty care visit because it is a higher level of care. The number of medication copays charged depends on the number of each 30-day supply or less of medication filled. Inpatient copays are based on both a standard charge for each 90 days of care within a 365-day period as well as a per diem (daily) charge. Together, the inpatient copay charges cover all services, including medications. With the exception of medication copays for outpatients, long-term care copays are a single, all-inclusive charge

## *Who qualifies for the annual cap on medication copays?*

The annual cap on medication copays applies to Veterans in Priority Groups 2 through 6 (Priority Group 1 is exempt from ALL copays). Because of their higher income, Veterans in Priority Groups 7 and 8 do NOT qualify for the medication copay annual cap. For those that qualify, once the annual limit is reached, all subsequent prescriptions filled during the calendar year will be free of the copay requirement.

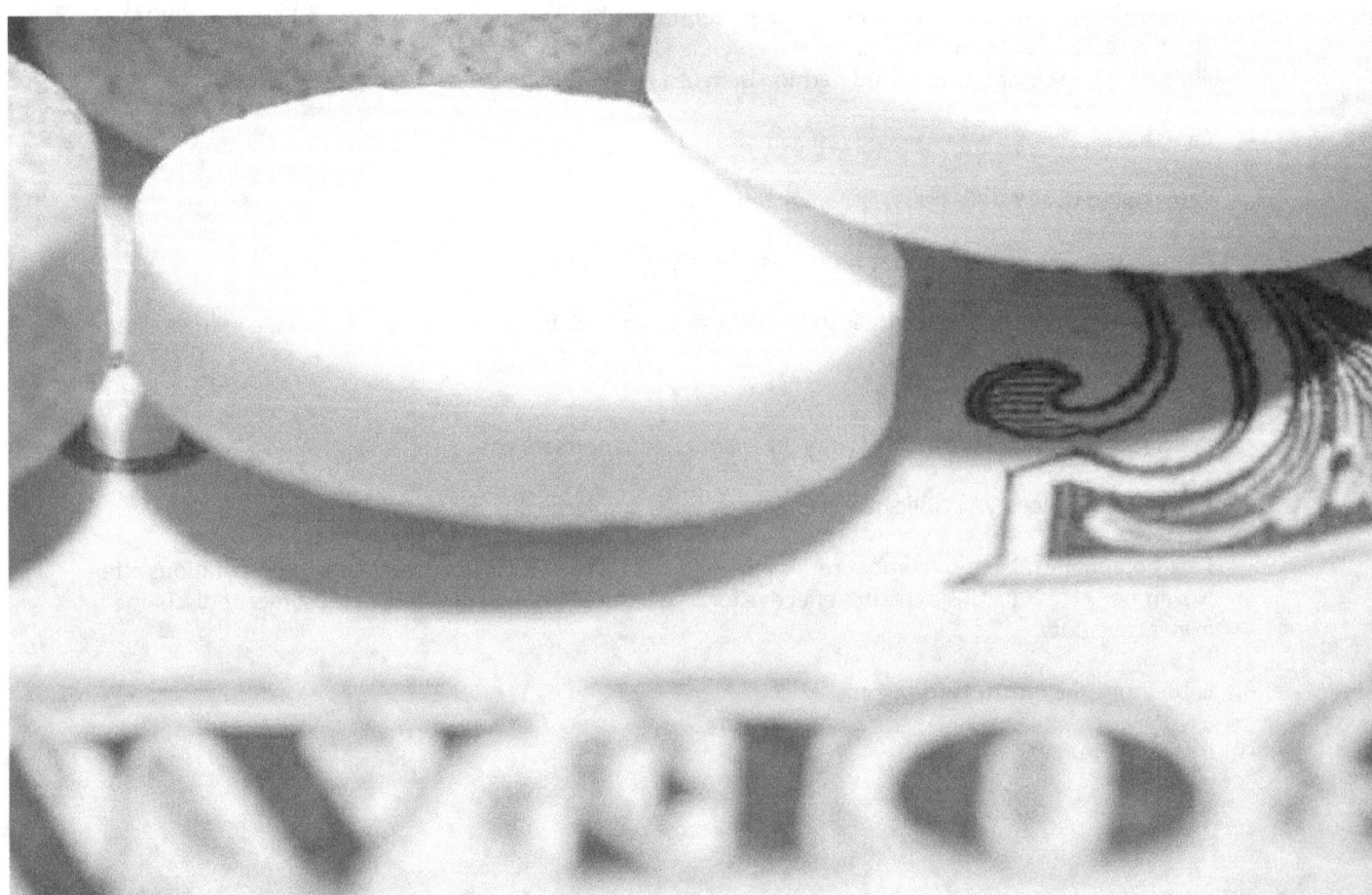

# Covered Services/Acute Care Benefits

**VA provides a robust Medical Benefits Package of health services that is available to all enrolled Veterans**

## Standard Benefits

### Preventive Care Services

- Immunizations
- Physical Examinations (including eye and hearing examinations)
- Health Care Assessments
- Screening Tests
- Health Education Programs

### Ambulatory (Outpatient) Diagnostic and Treatment Services

- Medical
- Surgical (including reconstructive/plastic surgery as a result of disease or trauma)
- Mental Health
- Substance Abuse

### Hospital (Inpatient) Diagnostic and Treatment Services

- Medical
- Surgical (including reconstructive/plastic surgery as a result of disease or trauma)
- Mental Health
- Substance Abuse

### Prescription Drugs (when prescribed by a VA physician)

## Limited Benefits

The following care services (partial listing) have limitations and may have special eligibility criteria:

- Ambulance Services
- Dental Care
- Eyeglasses
- Hearing Aids
- Home Health Care
- Maternity and Parturition (Childbirth) Services—usually provided in non-VA contracted hospitals at VA expense; care is limited to the mother and newborn. VA may furnish health care services to a newborn child of a woman Veteran who is receiving maternity care furnished by VA beginning with the date of birth plus the first seven calendar days after birth.
- Non-VA Health Care Services

# General Exclusions (partial listing)

- Abortions and abortion counseling
- Cosmetic surgery, except where determined by VA to be medically necessary for reconstructive or psychiatric care
- Gender alteration
- Health club or spa membership, even for rehabilitation
- In-vitro fertilization
- Drugs, biological and medical devices not approved by the Food and Drug Administration, unless part of formal clinical trial under an approved research program or when prescribed under a compassionate use exemption
- Medical care for a Veteran who is either a patient or inmate in an institution of another government agency if that agency has a duty to provide the care or services
- Services not ordered and provided by licensed/accredited professional staff
- Special private duty nursing

*Maternity and Parturition (Childbirth) Services— usually provided in non-VA contracted hospitals at VA expense; care is limited to the mother and newborn...*

## VA Foreign Medical Program (FMP)

A health care benefits program for U.S. Veterans with VA-rated service-connected conditions who are living or traveling abroad. Foreign benefits are administered by two separate offices, depending on where the health care services are obtained.

### Veterans in the Philippines

| Address | Phone | Fax |
|---|---|---|
| U.S. Department of Veterans Affairs Manila Outpatient Clinic 1501 Roxas Blvd 1302 Pasay City Philippines | 011-632-318-VETS (8387) | 011-632-310-5957 |

### All other countries

| Address | Telephone | Fax | Web site |
|---|---|---|---|
| Foreign Medical Program PO Box 469061 Denver CO 80246-9061 | 303-331-7590 | 303-331-7803 | www.va.gov/hac |
| To contact FMP online go to www.va.gov/hac/contact - *(see Foreign Medical Program)* | | | |

# Frequently Asked Questions

## *Hearing aids and eyeglasses are listed as "limited" benefits. Under what circumstances do I qualify?*

VA medical services include diagnostic audiology and diagnostic and preventive eye care services. VA will provide hearing aids and eyeglasses to Veteran's who receive increased pension based on the need for regular aid and attendance or being permanently housebound, receive compensation for a service-connected disability, are a former POW, were awarded a Purple Heart, currently enrolled in a Vocational Rehabilitation program, are about to be admitted to a VA Blind Rehabilitation Program, you have a eye or hearing impairment that resulted from the existence of another condition for which you are currently receiving VA care, or which resulted from treatment of the medical condition, or your vision or hearing are so severely impaired that aids are necessary to permit active participation in your own medical treatment. Otherwise, hearing aids and eyeglasses are provided only in special circumstances, and not for normally occurring hearing or vision loss. For additional information, contact the prosthetic representative of your local VA health care facility.

## *Am I eligible for dental care?*

Dental benefits are provided by the Department of Veterans Affairs (VA) according to law. In some instances, VA is authorized to provide extensive dental care, while in other cases treatment may be limited. The Chart below describes dental eligibility criteria and contains information to assist Veterans in understanding their eligibility for VA dental care.

The eligibility for outpatient dental care is not the same as for most other VA medical benefits and is categorized into classes. For instance, if you are eligible for VA dental care under Class I, IIC, or IV you are eligible for any necessary dental care to maintain or restore oral health and masticatory function, including repeat care. Other classes have time and/or service limitations.

| If you: | You are eligible for: | Through |
|---|---|---|
| Have a service-connected compensable dental disability or condition. | Any needed dental care. | Class I |
| Are a former prisoner of war. | Any needed dental care. | Class IIC |
| Have service-connected disabilities rated 100% disabling, or are unemployable and paid at the 100% rate due to service-connected conditions. | Any needed dental care.<br>*[Please note: Veterans paid at the 100% rate based on a temporary rating, such as extended hospitalization for a service-connected disability, convalescence or pre-stabilization are not eligible for comprehensive outpatient dental services based on this temporary rating]* | Class IV |
| Apply for dental care within 180 days of discharge or release from a period of active duty (under conditions other than dishonorable) of 90 days or more during the Persian Gulf War era | One-time dental care if your DD214 certificate of discharge does not indicate that a complete dental examination and all appropriate dental treatment had been rendered prior to discharge.* | Class II |
| Have a service-connected noncompensable dental condition or disability resulting from combat wounds or service trauma. | Needed care for the service-connected condition(s). A Dental Trauma Rating (VA Form 10-564-D) or VA Regional Office Rating Decision letter (VA Form 10-7131) identifies the tooth/teeth eligible for care. | Class IIA |

| | | |
|---|---|---|
| Have a dental condition clinically determined by VA to be associated with and aggravating a service-connected medical condition. | Dental care to treat the oral conditions that are determined by a VA dental professional to have a direct and material detrimental effect to your service connected medical condition. | Class III |
| Are actively engaged in a 38 USC Chapter 31 vocational rehabilitation program. | Dental care to the extent necessary as determined by a VA dental professional to:<br>• Make possible your entrance into a rehabilitation program<br>• Achieve the goals of your vocational rehabilitation program<br>• Prevent interruption of your rehabilitation program<br>• Hasten the return to a rehabilitation program if you are in interrupted or leave status<br>• Hasten the return to a rehabilitation program of a Veteran placed in discontinued status because of illness, injury or a dental condition, or<br>Secure and adjust to employment during the period of employment assistance, or enable you to achieve maximum independence in daily living. | Class V |
| Are receiving VA care or are scheduled for inpatient care and require dental care for a condition complicating a medical condition currently under treatment. | Dental care to treat the oral conditions that are determined by a VA dental professional to complicate your medical condition currently under treatment. | Class VI |
| Are an enrolled Veteran who may be homeless and receiving care under VHA Directive 2007-039. | A one-time course of dental care that is determined medically necessary to relieve pain, assist you to gain employment, or treat moderate, severe, or complicated and severe gingival and periodontal conditions. | Class IIB |

*\* Note: Public Law 83 enacted June 16, 1955, amended Veterans' eligibility for outpatient dental services. As a result, any Veteran who received a dental award letter from VBA dated before 1955 in which VBA determined the dental conditions to be noncompensable are no longer eligible for Class II outpatient dental treatment.*

Veterans receiving hospital, nursing home, or domiciliary care will be provided dental services that are professionally determined by a VA dentist, in consultation with the referring physician, to be essential to the management of the patient's medical condition under active treatment.

For more information about eligibility for VA medical and dental benefits, contact VA at 1-877-222-VETS (8387) or **www.va.gov/healthbenefits**.

## Am I limited to a specific number of inpatient days or outpatient visits during a given period of time?

For acute care services (inpatient days of care and outpatient visits), there are no limits.

## Do I qualify for routine health care at non-VA facilities at VA expense?

Generally no. To qualify for routine care at non-VA facilities at VA expense (otherwise known as **Fee Basis care**), you must first be given a written referral. Included among the factors in determining whether such care will be authorized is your medical condition and availability of VA services within your geographic area. VA copays may be applicable.

## Am I eligible for emergency care at a non-VA facility?

An eligible Veteran may receive emergency care at a non-VA health care facility at VA expense when a VA facility or other Federal health care facility with which VA has an agreement is unable to furnish economical care due to the Veteran's geographical inaccessibility to a VA medical facility, or when VA is unable to furnish the needed emergency services.

An emergency is defined as a condition of such a nature that a prudent layperson would have reasonably expected that delay in seeking immediate medical attention would have been hazardous to life or health. VA may directly refer or authorize the Veteran to receive emergency care at a non-VA facility at VA expense, or VA may pay for emergency care furnished certain Veterans by a non-VA facility without prior VA approval under certain conditions.

## Are there any payment limitations for non-VA emergency care?

Emergency care must be pre-authorized by VA. When the emergency care is not authorized in advance by VA, it may be considered as preauthorized care when the nearest VA medical facility is notified within 72 hours of admission, the Veteran is eligible, and the care rendered is emergent in nature. Claims for non-VA emergency care not authorized by VA in advance of services being furnished must be timely filed; because timely filing requirements differ by type of claim, you should contact the nearest VA medical facility as soon as possible to avoid payment denial for an untimely filed claim.

Payment may not be approved for any period beyond the date on which the medical emergency ended, except when VA cannot accommodate transfer of the Veteran to a VA or other Federal facility. An emergency is deemed to have ended at that point when a VA physician has determined that, based on sound medical judgment, a Veteran who received emergency hospital care could have been transferred from the non-VA facility to a VA medical center for continuation of treatment.

## What type of emergency care can VA authorize in advance?

| Subject to eligibility and payment limitations described at the top of page 29, VA may preauthorize and issue payment for non-VA emergency care when treatment is needed for: | Inpatient Care | Outpatient Care |
|---|:---:|:---:|
| The Veteran's VA rated service-connected disability, or for a nonservice-condition that is associated with and aggravating the Veteran's service-connected condition | ✓ | ✓ |
| A disability for which the Veteran was released from active duty | ✓ | ✓ |
| Any condition of a Veteran who is rated by VA as Permanently and Totally disabled due to a service connected disability | ✓ | ✓ |
| Any condition of a Veteran who is an active participant in the VA Chapter 31 Vocational Rehabilitation program, who needs treatment medically determined to make possible the Veteran's entrance into a course of training, or prevent interruption of a course of training which was interrupted due to such illness, injury, or dental condition. | ✓ | ✓ |
| Any condition for a Veteran who has a VA service-connected disability rating of 50% or greater | | ✓ |
| A condition for which the Veteran has been furnished VA hospital care, nursing home, domiciliary care, or medical services and who requires medical services to complete treatment incident to such care or services | | ✓ |
| Any condition of a Veteran who is in receipt of increased VA pension, or additional VA compensation or allowances based on the need for regular aid and attendance or by reason of being permanently housebound | | ✓ |
| Any condition for a Veteran of World War I | | ✓ |

| | | |
|---|---|---|
| A condition requiring emergency care that developed while the Veteran was receiving medical services in a VA facility or Contract Nursing Home or during VA authorized travel | ✓ | ✓ |
| Any condition that will obviate the need for hospital admission for a Veteran in the state of Alaska or Hawaii and US Territories, excluding Puerto Rico | | ✓ |
| Any condition for women Veterans. | ✓ | |
| Any dental services and treatment, and related dental appliances, for Veterans who are former prisoners of war | | ✓ |

## Can VA pay for non-VA emergency care that is not preauthorized?

VA has limited payment authority when emergency care at a non-VA facility is provided without authorization by VA in advance of services being furnished or notification to VA is not made within 72 hours of admission. VA may pay for unauthorized emergency care as indicated below. Since payment may be limited to the point your condition is stable for transfer to a VA facility, the nearest VA medical facility should be contacted as soon as possible for all care not authorized by VA in advance of the services being furnished.

| For service-connected Veterans | For nonservice-connected conditions |
|---|---|
| VA may only pay for emergency care provided in a non-VA facility for certain Veterans who are rated by VA with a service-connected disability. VA may pay for emergency inpatient or outpatient care when treatment is needed for: | VA may only pay for emergency care provided in a non-VA facility for treatment of a nonservice-connected condition only if **all** of the following conditions are met: |
| The Veteran's VA rated service connected disability, or for a nonservice-condition that is associated with and aggravating the Veteran's service-connected condition | The episode of care cannot be paid as an unauthorized claim for service-connected Veterans |
| A disability for which the Veteran was released from active duty | The Veteran is enrolled in the VHA health care system and received VA medical care within a 24 month period preceding the furnishing of the emergency treatment |
| Any condition of a Veteran who is rated by VA as Permanently and Totally disabled due to a service connected disability | The Veteran is personally liable to the health care provider for the emergency treatment which meets the prudent layperson definition of an emergency |
| Any condition of a Veteran who is an active participant in the VA Chapter 31 Vocational Rehabilitation program, | The Veteran is not entitled to care or services under a health plan contract |
| who needs treatment medically determined to make possible the Veteran's entrance into a course of training, or prevent interruption of a course of training which was interrupted due to such illness, injury, or dental condition | The Veteran has no other contractual or legal recourse against a third party that would, in whole, extinguish the Veteran's liability and the claim must be filed within 90 days from the date of discharge, or the date that the Veteran exhausted without success action to obtain payment from a third party. |

## Does VA offer compensation for travel expenses to and from a VA facility?

If you meet specific criteria (see Medically Related Travel Benefits on page 6), you are eligible for travel benefits. Travel benefits are subject to a deductible. Exceptions to the deductible requirement include: 1) travel for a compensation and pension examination; and 2) travel by an ambulance or a specially equipped van. Because travel benefits are subject to annual mileage rate and deductible changes, we publish a separate document detailing these amounts each year. You can obtain a copy at any VA health care facility.

# Long-Term Care Benefits

## Standard Benefits

The following long-term care services are available to all enrolled Veterans.

## Geriatric Evaluation

Geriatric evaluation is the comprehensive assessment of a Veteran's ability to care for him/herself, his/her physical health and social environment, which leads to a plan of care. The plan could include treatment, rehabilitation, health promotion and social services. These evaluations are performed by inpatient Geriatric Evaluation and Management (GEM) Units, GEM clinics, geriatric primary care clinics and other outpatient settings.

## Adult Day Health Care

The adult day health care (ADHC) program is a therapeutic day care program, providing medical and rehabilitation services to disabled Veterans in a combined setting.

## Respite Care

Respite care provides supportive care to Veterans on a short-term basis to give the caregiver a planned period of relief from the physical and emotional demands associated with providing care. Respite care can be provided in the home or other non institutional settings.

## Home Care

Skilled home care is provided by VA and contract agencies to Veterans that are homebound with chronic diseases and includes nursing, physical/occupational therapy and social services.

## Hospice/Palliative Care

Hospice/palliative care programs offer pain management, symptom control, and other medical services to terminally ill Veterans or Veterans in the late stages of the chronic disease process. Services also include respite care as well as bereavement counseling to family members.

NOTE: There are no copays for hospice care provided in any setting.

*For those Veterans who do not qualify for cost-free services, the financial assessment for long term care services is used to determine the copay requirement.*

## Financial Assessment for Long-Term Care Services

For Veterans who are not automatically exempt from making copays for long-term care services (see Copays on page 16), a separate financial assessment (VA Form 10-10EC, APPLICATION FOR EXTENDED CARE SERVICES) must be completed to determine whether they qualify for cost-free services or to what extent they are required to make long-term care copays. Unlike copays for other VA health care services, which are based on fixed charges for all, long-term care, copay charges are individually adjusted based on each Veteran's financial status.

## Limited Benefits

## VA Community Living Centers (VA Nursing Home) Programs

While some Veterans qualify for indefinite Community Living Center (formerly known as nursing home care) services, other Veterans may qualify for a limited period of time. Among those that automatically qualify for indefinite community living care are Veterans whose service-connected condition is clinically determined to require nursing home care and Veterans with a service-connected rating of 70% or more and unemployable. Other Veterans may be provided short-term community living care, if space and resources are available.

## Domiciliary Care

Domiciliary care provides rehabilitative and long-term, health maintenance care for Veterans who require some medical care, but who do not require all the services provided in nursing homes. Domiciliary care emphasizes rehabilitation and return to the community. VA may provide domiciliary care to Veterans whose annual income does not exceed the maximum annual rate of VA pension or to Veterans who have no adequate means of support.

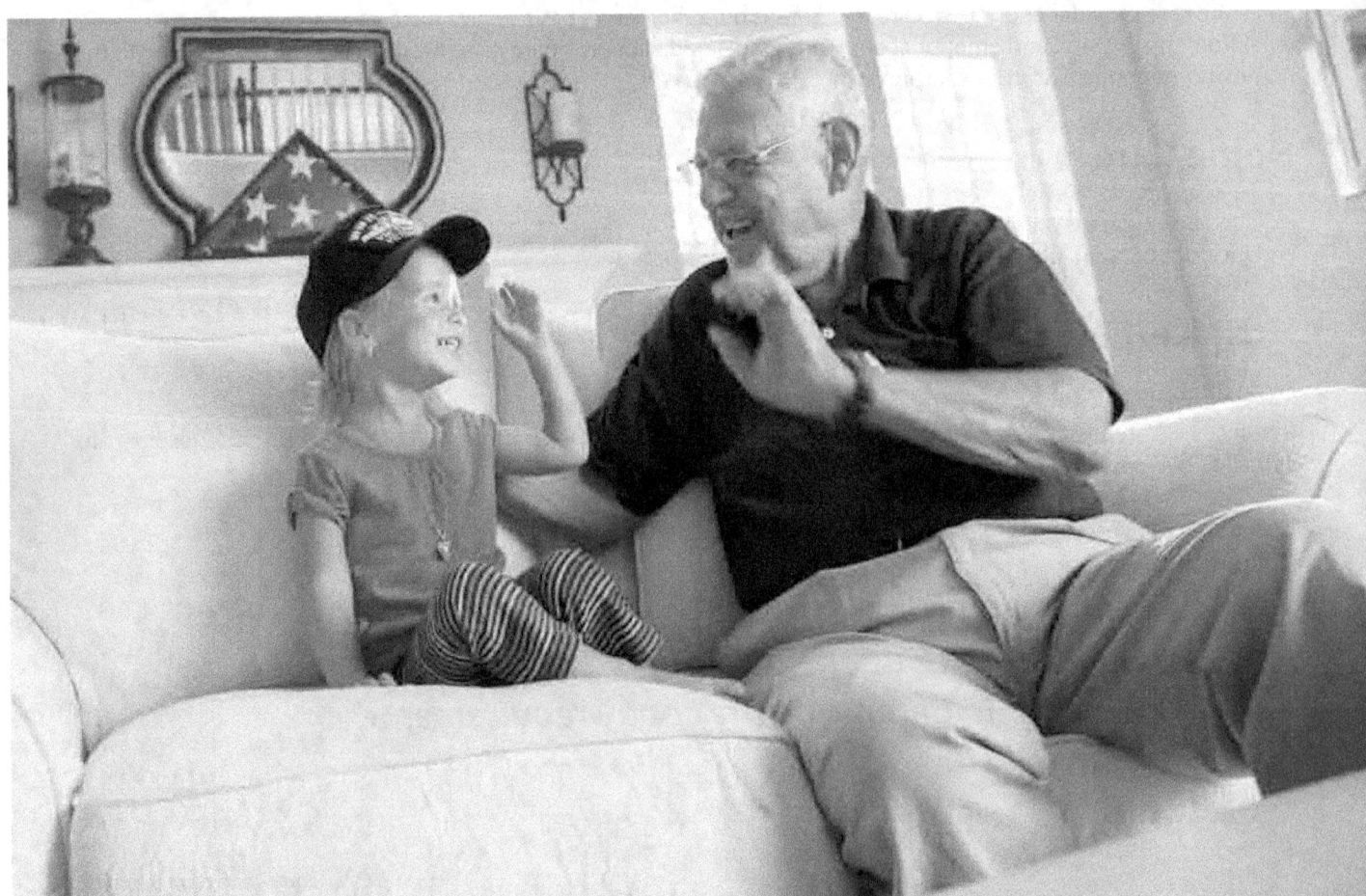

# Frequently Asked Questions

### *I already provided financial information on my initial VA application, why is it necessary to complete a separate financial assessment for long-term care?*

Unlike the information collected from the financial assessment, which is based on your previous year's income, the 10-10EC is designed to assess your current financial status, including current expenses. This in-depth analysis provides the necessary monthly income/expense information to determine whether you qualify for cost-free long-term care or a significant reduction from the maximum copay charge.

### *Once I submit a completed VA Form 10-10EC, who notifies me of my long-term care copay requirements?*

The social worker or case manager involved in your long-term care placement will provide you with an annual projection of your monthly copay charges.

### *Assuming I qualify for nursing home care, how is it determined whether the care will be provided in a VA facility or a private nursing home at VA expense?*

Generally, if you qualify for indefinite nursing home care, that care will be furnished in a VA facility. Care may be provided in a private facility under VA contract when there is compelling medical or social need. If you do not qualify for indefinite care, you may be placed in a community nursing home—generally not to exceed six months—following an episode of VA care. The purpose of this short-term placement is to provide assistance to you and your families while alternative, long-term arrangements are explored.

### *For Veterans who do not qualify for indefinite VA Community Living Center care at VA expense, what assistance is available for making alternative arrangements?*

When the need for nursing home care extends beyond the Veteran's eligibility, our social workers will help family members identify possible sources for financial assistance. Our staff will review basic Medicare and Medicaid eligibility and direct the family to the appropriate sources for further assistance, including possible application for additional VA benefit programs.

# Additional VA Health Benefits
## Dependents and Survivors

| CHAMPVA — a health care benefits program for: | | |
|---|---|---|
| Dependents of Veterans who have been rated by VA as having a service-connected total and permanent disability. | | |
| Survivors of Veterans who died from VA-rated service-connected condition(s), or who at the time of death, were rated permanently and totally disabled from a VA-rated service-connected condition(s). | | |
| Survivors of persons who died in the line of duty and not due to misconduct and not otherwise entitled to benefits under DoD's TRICARE program. | | |
| **Address** | **Telephone** | **Fax** |
| CHAMPVA<br>PO Box 469063<br>Denver CO 80246-9063 | 800-733-8387 | 303-331-7804 |
| To contact CHAMPVA online | **www.va.gov/hac/contact** (see CHAMPVA) | |
| Web site | **www.va.gov/hac** | |

| Children of Women Vietnam Veterans Health Care Benefits | |
|---|---|
| A program designed for women Vietnam Veterans' birth children who are determined by a VA Regional Office to have one or more covered birth defects. | |
| Address | Telephone |
| Children of Women Vietnam Veterans<br>PO Box 469065<br>Denver CO  80246-9065 | 888-820-1756 |
| | Fax |
| | 303-331-7807 |
| To contact CWVV online | Web site |
| **www.va.gov/hac/contact** (see CWVV) | **www.va.gov/hac** |

| Spina Bifida Health Care Benefits | |
|---|---|
| A program designed for certain birth children of Vietnam and Korea Veterans' birth children diagnosed with spina bifida and who are in receipt of a VA Regional Office award for spina bifida benefits. | |
| Address | Telephone |
| Spina Bifida Health Care<br>PO Box 469065<br>Denver CO  80246-9065 | 888-820-1756 |
| | Fax |
| | 303-331-7807 |
| To contact Spina Bifida online | Web site |
| **www.va.gov/hac/contact** (see Spina Bifida) | **www.va.gov/hac** |

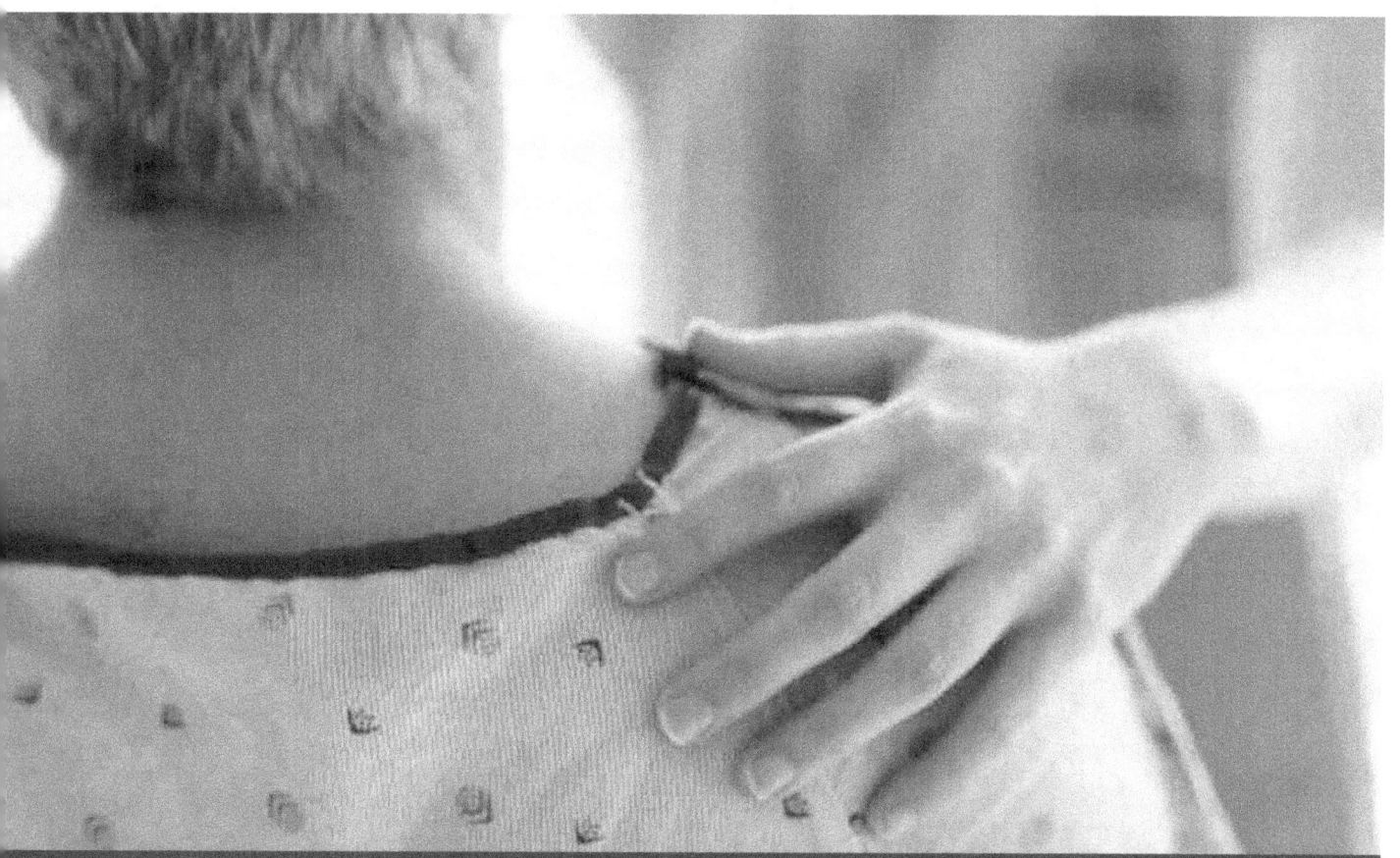

## Our Mission

**Our Servicemembers and Veterans have sacrificed to keep our country - and everything it represents - safe.  We honor and serve those men and women by fulfilling President Lincoln's promise** *"to care for him who shall have borne the battle, and for his widow, and his orphan."*

**We strive to provide Servicemembers and Veterans with the world-class benefits and services they have earned, and will adhere to the highest standards of compassion, commitment, excellence, professionalism, integrity, accountability, and stewardship.**

Thank you for your service.
Now let us serve you.